Copyright © 2023 by Monica Dimitrios

All rights reserved. No part of this publication may be reproduced, distributed, or transmitted in any form or by any means, including photocopying, recording, or other electronic or mechanical methods, without the prior written permission of the publisher, except in the case of brief quotations embodied in critical reviews and certain other noncommercial uses permitted by copyright law.

Table of Contents

Belly fat is more than a nuisance that makes your clothes feel tight.

Too much belly fat can increase your risk of certain chronic conditions. Drinking less alcohol, eating more protein, and lifting weights are just a few steps you can take to lose belly fat.

1. Avocado Hummus

Prep Time: 10 mins

Total Time: 10 mins

Servings: 10

Ingredients

- 1 (15 ounce) can no-salt-added chickpeas
- 1 ripe avocado, halved and pitted
- 1 cup fresh cilantro leaves
- ¼ cup tahini
- ¼ cup extra-virgin olive oil
- ¼ cup lemon juice
- 1 clove garlic
- 1 teaspoon ground cumin
- ½ teaspoon salt

Directions

1. Drain chickpeas, reserving 2 tablespoons of the liquid. Transfer the chickpeas and the reserved liquid to a food processor. Add avocado, cilantro, tahini, oil, lemon juice, garlic, cumin and salt. Puree until very smooth. Serve with veggie chips, pita chips or crudités.

2. Berry-Kefir Smoothie

Prep Time: 5 mins

Total Time: 5 mins

Servings: 1

Ingredients

- 1 ½ cups frozen mixed berries
- 1 cup plain kefir
- ½ medium banana
- 2 teaspoons almond butter
- ½ teaspoon vanilla extract

Directions

1. Combine berries, kefir, banana, almond butter and vanilla in a blender. Blend until smooth.

3. Avocado & Smoked Salmon Omelet

Prep Time: 10 mins

Total Time: 10 mins

Servings: 1

Ingredients

- 2 large eggs
- 1 teaspoon low-fat milk
- Pinch of salt
- 1 teaspoon extra-virgin olive oil plus 1/2 teaspoon, divided
- ¼ avocado, sliced
- 1 ounce smoked salmon
- 1 tablespoon chopped fresh basil

Directions

1. Beat eggs with milk and salt in a small bowl. Heat 1 teaspoon oil in a small nonstick skillet

over medium heat. Add the egg mixture and cook until the bottom is set and the center is still a bit runny, 1 to 2 minutes. Flip the omelet over and cook until set, about 30 seconds more. Transfer to a plate. Top with avocado, salmon and basil. Drizzle with the remaining 1/2 teaspoon oil.

4. Miso Soup Cup of Noodles with Shrimp & Green Tea Soba

Prep Time: 15 mins

Total Time: 25 mins

Servings: 3

Ingredients

- 4 tablespoons white miso

- 6 teaspoons mirin

- 3 teaspoons unseasoned rice vinegar

- 1 ½ cups diagonally sliced snow peas (about 5 ounces)

- 9 ounces peeled cooked shrimp

- 1 ½ teaspoons dried wakame

- 1 1/2 cups cooked green tea soba noodles (from 3-4 ounces dried)

- 3 tablespoons thinly sliced scallions

- 1 (3 inch) square dried kombu, snipped into 3 equal strips

- 3 cups very hot water, divided

Directions

1. Add 1 tablespoon plus 1 teaspoon miso, 2 teaspoons mirin and 1 teaspoon vinegar to each of three 1 1/2-pint canning jars. Layer 1/2 cup snow peas, 3 ounces shrimp, 1/2 teaspoon wakame and 1/2 cup noodles into each jar. Top each with 1 table-spoon scallions. Fit one piece of kombu between the ingredients and the side of each jar. Cover and refrigerate for up to 3 days.

2. To prepare each jar: Add 1 cup very hot water to the jar, cover and shake very well to dissolve the miso. Uncover and microwave on High in 1-minute increments until steaming hot, 2 to 3 minutes total. Discard the kombu. Stir to make sure the miso is dissolved. Let stand a few minutes before eating.

Prep Time: 15 mins

Total Time: 15 mins

Servings: 1

Ingredients

- 1 cup cooked quinoa
- ⅓ cup canned chickpeas, rinsed and drained
- ½ cup cucumber slices
- ½ cup cherry tomatoes, halved
- ¼ avocado, diced
- 3 tablespoons hummus
- 1 tablespoon finely chopped roasted red pepper
- 1 tablespoon lemon juice
- 1 tablespoon water, plus more if desired
- 1 teaspoon chopped fresh parsley
- Pinch of salt
- Pinch of ground pepper

Directions

1. Arrange quinoa, chickpeas, cucumbers, tomatoes and avocado in a wide bowl.

2. Stir hummus, roasted red pepper, lemon juice and water in a bowl. Add more water to reach desired consistency for dressing. Add parsley, salt and pepper and stir to combine. Serve with the Buddha bowl.

6. Sweet Potato-Peanut Bisque

Total Time: 30 mins

Servings: 5

Ingredients

- 2 large sweet potatoes (10-12 ounces each)

- 1 tablespoon canola oil

- 1 small yellow onion, chopped

- 1 large clove garlic, minced

- 3 cups reduced-sodium tomato-vegetable juice blend or tomato juice

- 1 (4 ounce) can diced green chiles, preferably hot, drained

- 2 teaspoons minced fresh ginger

- 1 teaspoon ground allspice

- 1 (15 ounce) can vegetable broth

- ½ cup smooth natural peanut butter

- Freshly ground pepper to taste

- Chopped fresh cilantro leaves for garnish

Directions

1. Prick sweet potatoes in several places with a fork. Microwave on High until just cooked through, 7 to 10 minutes. Set aside to cool.

2. Meanwhile, heat oil in a large saucepan or Dutch oven over medium-high heat. Add onion and cook, stirring, until it just begins to brown, 2 to 4 minutes. Add garlic and cook, stirring, for 1 minute more. Stir in juice, green chiles, ginger and allspice. Adjust the heat so the mixture boils gently; cook for 10 minutes.

3. Meanwhile, peel the sweet potatoes and chop into bite-size pieces. Add half to the pot. Place the other half in a food processor or blender along with broth and peanut butter. Puree until completely smooth. Add the puree to the pot and stir well to combine. Thin the bisque with water, if desired. Season with pepper. Heat until hot. Garnish with cilantro, if desired.

Prep Time: 30 mins

Total Time: 30 mins

Servings: 4

Ingredients

- 1 medium sweet potato, peeled if desired, cut into 1-inch chunks
- 3 tablespoons extra-virgin olive oil, divided
- ½ teaspoon salt, divided
- ½ teaspoon ground pepper, divided
- 2 tablespoons tahini
- 2 tablespoons water
- 1 tablespoon lemon juice
- 1 small clove garlic, minced
- 2 cups cooked quinoa
- 1 15-ounce can chickpeas, rinsed
- 1 firm ripe avocado, diced
- ¼ cup chopped fresh cilantro or parsley

Directions

1. Preheat oven to 425 degrees F.

2. Toss sweet potato with 1 tablespoon oil and 1/4 teaspoon each salt and pepper in a medium bowl. Transfer to a rimmed baking sheet. Roast, stirring once, until tender, 15 to 18 minutes.

3. Meanwhile, whisk the remaining 2 tablespoons oil, tahini, water, lemon juice, garlic and the remaining 1/4 teaspoon each salt and pepper in a small bowl.

4. To serve, divide quinoa among 4 bowls. Top with equal amounts of sweet potato, chickpeas and avocado. Drizzle with the tahini sauce. Sprinkle with parsley (or cilantro).

Prep Time: 25 mins

Total Time: 50 mins

Servings: 2

Ingredients

Rice

- 1 ¼ cups water
- ½ cup brown basmati rice
- ¼ cup raisins
- 1 teaspoon extra-virgin olive oil
- 1 teaspoon onion powder or garlic powder
- ½ teaspoon ground turmeric or 1 teaspoon freshly grated turmeric
- ¼ teaspoon ground cinnamon
- ¼ teaspoon ground black pepper
- ⅛ teaspoon kosher salt

Vegetables & Chickpeas

- 2 tablespoons coconut oil or ghee
- 1 (15 ounce) can chickpeas, rinsed and patted dry
- 1 teaspoon garam masala or Indian curry powder
- 1 cup roasted root vegetables (see associated recipe)
- 1 teaspoon sugar or honey
- ¼ teaspoon kosher salt
- ¼ teaspoon ground pepper
- 2 tablespoons lemon juice
- 2 tablespoons low-fat plain yogurt or tahini

Directions

1. To prepare rice: Combine water, rice, raisins, olive oil, onion powder (or garlic powder), turmeric, cinnamon, pepper and 1/8 teaspoon salt in a small saucepan. Bring to a boil. Cover, reduce heat to maintain a gentle simmer and

cook until the liquid is absorbed, 35 to 40 minutes. Remove from heat and let stand, covered, for 10 minutes.

2. Meanwhile, to prepare vegetables & chickpeas: Heat coconut oil (or ghee) in a medium skillet over medium heat. Add chickpeas and cook, stirring, until crispy, 3 to 5 minutes. Stir in garam masala (or curry powder) and cook until fragrant, about 1 minute. Add roasted root vegetables, sugar (or honey), salt and pepper; cook, stirring often, until heated through, 2 to 4 minutes. Stir in lemon juice.

3. Serve the vegetable mixture over the rice, topped with yogurt (or tahini). Garnish with herbs, if desired.

Total Time: 50 mins

Servings: 8

Ingredients

- 4 large lemons, divided, plus more for garnish
- 8 large artichokes
- 2 cups water
- 6 cloves garlic, chopped
- ¼ cup chopped fresh dill, plus more for garnish
- 1 teaspoon salt
- ¼ teaspoon ground pepper
- 1 ½ tablespoons extra-virgin olive oil

Directions

1. Squeeze the juice from 2 lemons. Fill a large bowl of cold water and add the juice and rinds.

Use a paring knife to trim the bottom 1/4 inch off the artichoke stems. Snip the thorn off the leaves with kitchen shears. Cut off about 1 inch from the tops. With a melon baller or spoon, scoop out the fuzzy chokes. Place the trimmed artichokes in the lemon water to prevent discoloration.

2. Squeeze 1/3 cup juice from the remaining 2 lemons. Combine the juice with 2 cups water in a large nonreactive pot wide enough to hold the artichokes in a single layer. Drain the artichokes and lay them on their sides in the pot. Top with garlic, dill, salt and pepper. Bring to a boil. Reduce heat to low, cover and simmer, turning the artichokes once, until tender when pierced with a fork, 18 to 20 minutes.

3. With a slotted spoon, transfer the artichokes to a deep platter. Simmer the liquid remaining in the pan over medium-high heat until reduced to 1 1/4 cups, about 10 minutes; spoon over the artichokes. Let cool to room temperature.

4. To serve, drizzle the artichokes with oil and baste with sauce. Garnish with chopped dill and lemon wedges, if desired.

Prep Time: 10 mins

Total Time: 10 mins

Servings: 8

Ingredients

- 1 (15 ounce) can no-salt-added chickpeas
- ¼ cup tahini
- ¼ cup extra-virgin olive oil
- ¼ cup lemon juice
- 1 clove garlic
- 1 teaspoon ground cumin
- ½ teaspoon chili powder
- ½ teaspoon salt

Directions

1. Drain chickpeas, reserving 1/4 cup of the liquid. Transfer the chickpeas and the reserved

liquid to a food processor. Add tahini, oil, lemon juice, garlic, cumin, chili powder and salt. Puree until very smooth, 2 to 3 minutes.

Total Time: 10 mins

Servings: 1

Ingredients

- ¼ cup boiling water
- 1 teaspoon matcha tea powder
- 1 cup low-fat milk
- 1 teaspoon honey

Directions

1. Blend boiling water with matcha powder in a blender until foamy. Heat milk with honey until almost boiling. Vigorously whisk the milk until frothy. Pour the milk into a mug, then pour in the tea.

12. Whole-Wheat Veggie Wrap

Prep Time: 10 mins

Total Time: 10 mins

Servings: 1

Ingredients

- 1 8-inch whole-wheat tortilla
- 2 tablespoons hummus
- ¼ avocado, mashed
- 1 cup sliced fresh vegetables of your choice
- 2 tablespoons shredded sharp Cheddar cheese

Directions

1. Lay tortilla on work surface. Spread hummus and avocado on the tortilla. Add veggies and Cheddar and roll up. Cut in half before serving.

Total Time: 10 mins

Servings: 16

Ingredients

- 1 large bunch fresh basil
- 2 ripe avocados
- ½ cup walnuts or hemp seeds
- 2 tablespoons lemon juice
- 3 cloves garlic
- ½ teaspoon fine sea salt
- ½ cup extra-virgin olive oil
- Ground pepper to taste

Directions

1. Strip basil leaves from the stems and add to a food processor along with avocados, walnuts (or hemp seeds), lemon juice, garlic and salt;

pulse until finely chopped. Add oil and process to form a thick paste. Season with pepper.

14. Peanut Noodles with Shredded Chicken &
Vegetables

Total Time: 30 mins

Servings: 6

Ingredients

- 1 pound boneless, skinless chicken breasts

- ½ cup smooth natural peanut butter

- 2 tablespoons reduced-sodium soy sauce

- 2 teaspoons minced garlic

- 1 1/2 teaspoons chile-garlic sauce, or to taste

- 1 teaspoon minced fresh ginger

- 8 ounces whole-wheat spaghetti

- 1 12-ounce bag fresh vegetable medley, such as
  carrots, broccoli, snow peas

Directions

1. Put a large pot of water on to boil for cooking
   pasta.

2. Meanwhile, place chicken in a skillet or saucepan and add enough water to cover; bring to a boil. Cover, reduce heat to low and simmer gently until cooked through and no longer pink in the middle, 10 to 12 minutes. Transfer the chicken to a cutting board. When cool enough to handle, shred into bite-size strips.

3. Whisk peanut butter, soy sauce, garlic, chile-garlic sauce and ginger in a large bowl.

4. Cook pasta in the boiling water until not quite tender, about 1 minute less than specified in the package directions. Add vegetables and cook until the pasta and vegetables are just tender, 1 minute more. Drain, reserving 1 cup of the cooking liquid. Rinse the pasta and vegetables with cool water to refresh. Stir the reserved cooking liquid into the peanut sauce; add the pasta, vegetables and chicken; toss well to coat. Serve warm or chilled.

Total Time: 20 mins

Servings: 6

Ingredients

Creamy Dill Ranch Dressing

- 1 small shallot, peeled
- ¾ cup nonfat cottage cheese
- ¼ cup reduced-fat mayonnaise
- 2 tablespoons buttermilk powder
- 2 tablespoons white-wine vinegar
- ¼ cup nonfat milk
- 1 tablespoon chopped dill
- ¼ teaspoon salt
- ¼ teaspoon freshly ground pepper

Chickpea Salad

- 1 7-ounce can chickpeas, rinsed
- 3 cups peeled, seeded and diced cucumber

- 2 cups halved grape tomatoes or cherry tomatoes
- ¼ cup crumbled reduced-fat feta cheese
- ¼ cup diced red onion
- ½ cup Creamy Dill Ranch Dressing
- Freshly ground pepper to taste

Directions

1. To prepare dressing: With the food processor running, add shallot through the feed tube and process until finely chopped. Add cottage cheese, mayonnaise, buttermilk powder and vinegar. Process until smooth, scraping down the sides as necessary, about 3 minutes. Pour in milk while the processor is running. Scrape down the sides. Add dill, salt and pepper and process until combined. (Makes 1 1/4 cups.)
2. To prepare salad: Combine chickpeas, cucumber, tomatoes, cheese and onion in a medium bowl. Add dressing and pepper and

toss to coat. (Refrigerate extra dressing for up to 1 week.)

Total Time: 1 hr 30 mins

Servings: 4

Ingredients

- 3 cloves garlic, divided
- 3 pounds ripe plum tomatoes, cut into 1/2-inch pieces
- 1 medium onion, finely chopped
- 4 tablespoons extra-virgin olive oil, divided
- 2 tablespoons chopped fresh parsley, plus more for garnish
- ¾ teaspoon salt, divided
- ½ teaspoon ground pepper, divided
- 2 large green chiles, such as Anaheim, finely chopped
- 1 teaspoon ground cumin
- ⅓ cup chopped fresh basil
- 4 large eggs

- ½ cup crumbled feta cheese

- Hot sauce for serving

Directions

1. Preheat oven to 450°F.

2. Slice 2 garlic cloves. Toss with tomatoes, onion, 3 tablespoons oil, parsley and 1/4 teaspoon each salt and pepper in a large bowl. Spread evenly on a large rimmed baking sheet or in a shallow roasting pan. Roast until the tomatoes are shriveled and browned, about 45 minutes.

3. Chop the remaining garlic clove. Heat the remaining 1 tablespoon oil in a large skillet over medium heat. Add the garlic and chiles; cook, stirring, for 2 minutes. Add cumin and cook, stirring, for 30 seconds. Stir in the tomato mixture, the remaining 1/2 teaspoon salt and basil. Bring to a simmer and cook, stirring occasionally, until the tomatoes are mostly broken down, 6 to 8 minutes.

4. Make 4 deep indentations in the sauce with the back of a spoon and carefully crack an egg into each. Sprinkle the eggs with the remaining 1/4 teaspoon pepper. Cover and cook over medium-low until the whites are set, 6 to 8 minutes.

5. Remove from heat, sprinkle with feta and let stand, covered, for 2 minutes. (The eggs will continue to cook a bit as they stand.) Garnish with parsley and serve with hot sauce, if desired.

Prep Time: 10 mins

Total Time: 10 mins

Servings: 1

Ingredients

- 1 cup mixed salad greens
- 1 teaspoon red-wine vinegar
- 1 teaspoon extra-virgin olive oil
- Pinch of salt
- Pinch of pepper
- 2 slices sprouted whole-wheat bread, toasted
- ¼ cup plain hummus
- ¼ cup alfalfa sprouts
- ¼ avocado, sliced
- 2 teaspoons unsalted sunflower seeds

Directions

1. Toss greens with vinegar, oil, salt and pepper in a medium bowl. Spread each slice of toast with 2 tablespoons hummus. Top with sprouts, avocado and the greens and sprinkle with sunflower seeds.

Total Time: 20 mins

Servings: 4

Ingredients

- ⅓ cup creamy natural peanut butter
- ½ cup water, divided
- 2 tablespoons brown sugar
- 2 tablespoons reduced-sodium soy sauce, divided
- 1 tablespoon rice vinegar
- 2 tablespoons canola oil
- 1 ½ pounds broccoli crowns, trimmed and cut into 1-inch pieces
- 1 large red bell pepper, sliced
- 2 cloves garlic, minced
- 1/4-1/2 teaspoon crushed red pepper, or to taste
- ¼ cup chopped unsalted peanuts

Directions

1. Whisk peanut butter, 1/4 cup water, brown sugar, 1 tablespoon soy sauce and vinegar in a medium bowl until smooth. Set aside.

2. Heat oil in a wok or large skillet over medium heat. Add broccoli and cook, stirring frequently, until beginning to soften and brown in spots, about 6 minutes.

3. Add the remaining 1/4 cup water and 1 tablespoon soy sauce to the pan along with bell pepper and garlic. Cook, stirring frequently, until the pepper has softened and the liquid has evaporated, 2 to 4 minutes. Remove from the heat; stir in the reserved peanut sauce and season with crushed red pepper. Garnish with peanuts.

18. Chickpea Burgers & Tahini Sauce

Total Time: 25 mins

Servings: 4

Ingredients

- Chickpea burgers
- 1 19-ounce can chickpeas, rinsed
- 4 scallions, trimmed and sliced
- 1 egg
- 2 tablespoons all-purpose flour
- 1 tablespoon chopped fresh oregano
- ½ teaspoon ground cumin
- ¼ teaspoon salt
- 2 tablespoons extra-virgin olive oil
- 2 6-1/2-inch whole-wheat pitas, halved and warmed, if desired

Tahini sauce

- ½ cup low-fat plain yogurt

- 2 tablespoons tahini
- 1 tablespoon lemon juice
- ⅓ cup chopped flat-leaf parsley
- ¼ teaspoon salt

Directions

1. Place chickpeas, scallions, egg, flour, oregano, cumin and salt in a food processor. Pulse, stopping once or twice to scrape down the sides, until a coarse mixture forms that holds together when pressed. (The mixture will be moist.) Form into 4 patties.

2. Heat oil in a large nonstick skillet over medium-high heat. Add patties and cook until golden and beginning to crisp, 4 to 5 minutes. Carefully flip and cook until golden brown, 2 to 4 minutes more.

3. To prepare sauce & serve: Meanwhile, combine yogurt, tahini, lemon juice, parsley and salt in a medium bowl. Warm pitas, if desired

Prep Time: 25 mins

Total Time: 30 mins

Servings: 4

Ingredients

- 1 tablespoon extra-virgin olive oil
- 1 ½ cups chopped yellow onion
- 1 cup chopped red bell pepper
- ¾ cup chopped poblano pepper
- 1 tablespoon finely chopped jalapeño
- 1 tablespoon minced garlic
- ½ teaspoon ground cumin
- 2 tablespoons all-purpose flour
- 1 cup unsalted chicken broth
- 2 ounces reduced-fat cream cheese, at room temperature
- 2 cups chopped cooked chicken breast

- 1 (10 ounce) can no-salt-added diced tomatoes with green chiles, drained
- 2 (6 inch) corn tortillas, torn into pieces
- ¼ teaspoon salt
- ½ cup shredded Mexican-blend cheese
- 2 tablespoons chopped fresh cilantro

Directions

1. Preheat broiler to high.
2. Heat oil in a medium ovenproof skillet over medium-high heat until shimmering. Add onion, bell pepper, poblano and jalapeño; cook, stirring occasionally, until softened, 7 to 9 minutes. Add garlic and cumin; cook, stirring constantly, until fragrant, about 1 minute. Sprinkle flour over the vegetables and cook, stirring constantly, until they are thoroughly coated, about 1 minute.

3. Add broth and bring to a boil, stirring to combine. Cook, stirring, until slightly thickened, about 1 minute. Stir in cream cheese until melted. Stir in chicken, tomatoes, tortilla pieces and salt. Sprinkle evenly with cheese.

4. Place the skillet under the broiler and broil until the cheese is melted and browned, 1 to 2 minutes. Sprinkle with cilantro.

Prep Time: 25 mins

Total Time: 40 mins

Servings: 6

Ingredients

- 2 tablespoons olive oil
- 1 cup fresh or frozen corn kernels
- ½ cup diced green bell pepper
- ½ cup diced red bell pepper
- ½ cup diced onion
- 1 5-ounce package baby spinach
- 2 ½ cups shredded cooked chicken breast
- 1 8-ounce pouch red or green enchilada sauce, such as Frontera
- 1 ¼ cups prepared fresh salsa
- 8 5- or 6-inch corn tortillas, cut into 1-inch-thick strips
- 1 ½ cups shredded reduced-fat Cheddar cheese

- 1 cup coarsely chopped grape tomatoes
- ¼ cup chopped fresh cilantro
- ¼ cup matchstick-cut radishes

Directions

1. Preheat oven to 350°F.
2. Heat oil in a large ovenproof skillet, such as cast-iron. Add corn, green and red peppers, and onion; cook, stirring occasionally, until charred, 7 to 10 minutes. Gradually add spinach in batches; cook, stirring frequently, until wilted, 1 to 2 minutes.
3. Stir in chicken, enchilada sauce, and salsa until combined. Gently stir in tortilla strips. Sprinkle with cheese. Transfer to the oven and bake until bubbly, about 15 minutes.
4. Top the casserole with tomatoes, cilantro, and radishes.

21. Chicken & Broccoli Casserole

Prep Time: 20 mins

Total Time: 30 mins

Servings: 8

Ingredients

- 1 tablespoon canola oil
- 1 ½ pounds boneless, skinless chicken breasts, trimmed and cut into bite-size pieces
- 1 small onion, finely chopped
- ⅓ cup all-purpose flour
- 4 cups reduced-fat milk
- 3 cups broccoli florets
- 2 tablespoons water
- 2 (9 ounce) packages precooked brown rice
- 1 ½ cups shredded reduced-fat sharp Cheddar cheese
- 1 teaspoon dry mustard
- ½ teaspoon garlic powder

- ¾ teaspoon salt
- ½ teaspoon ground pepper
- 1 cup prepared crispy fried onions

Directions

1. Preheat oven to 400°F.
2. Heat oil in a large high-sided ovenproof skillet over medium-high heat. Add chicken and chopped onion; cook, stirring occasionally, until the chicken is no longer pink on the outside, about 7 minutes. Sprinkle the mixture with flour and cook, stirring occasionally, for 1 minute. Add milk to the pan and bring to a boil, stirring frequently. (Be careful, the pan will be very full.) Boil, stirring, for 1 minute.
3. Meanwhile, place broccoli and water in a microwave-safe container. Cover and microwave on High until the broccoli is tender, about 3 minutes. Drain.

4. Remove the pan from the heat and carefully stir in rice, cheese, dry mustard, garlic powder, salt, pepper and the broccoli. Sprinkle with crispy onions.

5. Bake the casserole until bubbling at the edges, about 10 minutes. Let stand for 5 minutes before serving.

Prep Time: 25 mins

Total Time: 50 mins

Servings: 6

Ingredients

- 8 ounces whole-wheat rotini
- 4 tablespoons extra-virgin olive oil, divided
- 1 cup chopped onion
- 1 (28 ounce) can no-salt-added crushed tomatoes
- 1 teaspoon garlic powder
- ½ teaspoon dried basil
- ½ teaspoon dried oregano
- ½ teaspoon salt
- ¼ teaspoon crushed red pepper
- 2 cups shredded cooked chicken
- 1 cup shredded mozzarella cheese
- ½ cup panko breadcrumbs

- ¼ cup grated Parmesan cheese
- 2 tablespoons chopped parsley

Directions

1. Preheat oven to 400 degrees F. Lightly coat an 8-inch-square baking dish with cooking spray.

2. Bring a large saucepan of water to a boil. Add rotini and cook according to package directions. Drain.

3. Meanwhile, heat 2 tablespoons oil in a large skillet over medium heat. Add onion and cook, stirring, until starting to soften, about 3 minutes. Add tomatoes, garlic powder, basil, oregano, salt and crushed red pepper; bring to a simmer. Cook, stirring, until thickened, about 5 minutes. Stir in chicken and the cooked rotini. Transfer to the prepared baking dish and top with mozzarella.

4. Stir panko, Parmesan, parsley and the remaining 2 tablespoons oil together in a small

bowl. Sprinkle over the casserole. Bake until hot and the topping is golden, 25 to 30 minutes.

23. Stuffed Cabbage Soup

Prep Time: 20 mins

Total Time: 1 hr

Servings: 8

Ingredients

- 2 tablespoons canola oil
- 1 ½ pounds lean ground beef
- 4 cups chopped green cabbage
- 2 cups chopped yellow onion
- 1 ¼ cups chopped carrots
- 1 cup chopped celery
- 2 tablespoons light brown sugar
- 1 tablespoon smoked paprika
- 1 teaspoon salt
- ½ teaspoon ground pepper
- ¼ teaspoon cayenne pepper
- 1 (15 ounce) can no-salt-added tomato sauce
- 4 cups unsalted chicken broth

- ¼ cup medium-grain brown rice
- 2 tablespoons chopped fresh flat-leaf parsley

Directions

1. Heat oil in a large heavy pot over medium-high heat. Add ground beef; cook, stirring often, until the meat is cooked through and starting to brown slightly, 6 to 7 minutes. Add cabbage, onion, carrots and celery; cook, stirring often, until the onion is translucent, about 5 minutes.

2. Add brown sugar, paprika, salt, pepper and cayenne to the beef mixture; cook over medium-high heat, stirring constantly, until the spices are toasted, about 1 minute. Stir in tomato sauce and broth, scraping the bottom of the pot with a wooden spoon to release any browned bits. Bring the soup to a boil over medium-high heat. Stir in rice. Reduce heat to low; cover and cook until the rice is tender, 30 to 35 minutes. If desired, sprinkle with parsley before serving.

Total Time: 25 mins

Servings: 6

Ingredients

- 2 teaspoons extra-virgin olive oil
- 2 leeks, white and light green parts only, cut into 1/4-inch rounds
- 1 tablespoon chopped fresh sage, or 1/4 teaspoon dried
- 2 14-ounce cans reduced-sodium chicken broth
- 2 cups water
- 1 15-ounce can cannellini beans, rinsed
- 1 2-pound roasted chicken, skin discarded, meat removed from bones and shredded (4 cups)

Directions

1. Heat oil in a Dutch oven over medium-high heat. Add leeks and cook, stirring often, until soft, about 3 minutes. Stir in sage and continue cooking until aromatic, about 30 seconds. Stir in broth and water, increase heat to high, cover and bring to a boil. Add beans and chicken and cook, uncovered, stirring occasionally, until heated through, about 3 minutes. Serve hot.

25. Breakfast Peanut Butter-Chocolate Chip Oatmeal Cakes

Prep Time: 15 mins

Total Time: 50 mins

Servings: 12

Ingredients

- 3 cups old-fashioned rolled oats
- 1 ½ cups low-fat milk
- ½ cup creamy natural peanut butter, divided
- ¼ cup unsweetened applesauce
- 2 large eggs, lightly beaten
- 3 tablespoons packed light brown sugar
- 1 teaspoon baking powder
- 1 teaspoon vanilla extract
- ½ teaspoon salt
- ¼ cup mini semisweet chocolate chips

Directions

1. Preheat oven to 375°F. Coat a 12-cup muffin tin with cooking spray.

2. Combine oats, milk, 1/4 cup peanut butter, applesauce, eggs, brown sugar, baking powder, vanilla and salt in a large bowl. Fill each muffin cup with a heaping 2 tablespoons of batter, then divide the remaining 1/4 cup peanut butter and chocolate chips among the muffin cups, about 1 teaspoon each. Cover with the remaining batter, about 2 tablespoons each. Bake until a toothpick inserted in the center comes out clean, about 25 minutes. Cool in the pan for 10 minutes, then turn out onto a wire rack. Serve warm or at room temperature.

26. Minestra Maritata Italian Wedding Soup

Prep Time: 20 mins

Total Time: 20 mins

Servings: 6

Ingredients

- 4 tablespoons extra-virgin olive oil, divided
- 1 ⅓ cups chopped yellow onion
- ⅔ cup chopped carrot
- ⅔ cup chopped celery
- 2 tablespoons minced garlic
- 6 cups unsalted chicken broth
- 6 ounces orzo, preferably whole-wheat
- 1 ½ tablespoons chopped fresh oregano
- ½ teaspoon kosher salt
- 24 cooked chicken meatballs (12 ounces), such as Easy Chicken Meatballs (see associated recipe)
- 4 cups baby spinach

- ¼ cup grated Parmesan cheese

Directions

1. Heat 1 tablespoon oil in a large pot over medium-high heat. Add onion, carrot, celery and garlic; cook, stirring occasionally, until the onion is translucent, 4 to 5 minutes.
2. Add broth, cover and bring to a boil. Add orzo, oregano and salt; cover and cook, stirring occasionally, until the orzo is just tender, about 9 minutes.
3. Stir in meatballs and spinach; cook until the meatballs are heated through and the spinach is wilted, 2 to 4 minutes.
4. Serve sprinkled with cheese and drizzled with the remaining 3 tablespoons oil.

Prep Time: 25 mins

Total Time: 25 mins

Servings: 6

Ingredients

- 6 ounces whole-wheat shell pasta
- 1 tablespoon canola oil
- ½ cup chopped onion
- 1 teaspoon brown sugar
- ½ cup chopped green bell pepper
- ½ cup chopped red bell pepper
- 1 pound ground chicken
- ½ teaspoon garlic powder
- ½ teaspoon onion powder
- ½ teaspoon ground pepper
- ¼ teaspoon salt
- 4 ounces cream cheese
- 2 teaspoons hot sauce

- 1 teaspoon Worcestershire sauce
- ½ cup shredded low-moisture, part-skim mozzarella cheese, divided
- 4 (1 ounce) slices provolone cheese

Directions

1. Bring a large pot of water to a boil. Cook pasta according to package directions. Reserve 1/2 cup of the cooking water, then drain the pasta.
2. Meanwhile, heat oil in a 12-inch cast-iron or other ovenproof skillet over medium-low heat. Add onion and cook until softened, 3 to 6 minutes. Add brown sugar; cook, stirring constantly, until the onion is golden brown, 6 to 8 minutes. Add green and red bell pepper; cook until tender, about 5 minutes. Increase heat to medium-high. Add chicken, garlic powder, onion powder, pepper and salt; cook until lightly browned, about 5 minutes.

Remove from heat. Add cream cheese, hot sauce, Worcestershire and 1/4 cup mozzarella, stir until melted and combined. Stir in the pasta and the reserved 1/2 cup pasta water. Top with provolone and the remaining 1/4 cup mozzarella.

3. Place oven rack in top third of oven and turn broiler to high. Broil the casserole until the cheeses are melted and golden, 3 to 4 minutes.

Prep Time: 20 mins

Total Time: 20 mins

Servings: 4

Ingredients

- 1 ½ tablespoons extra-virgin olive oil
- ½ cup panko breadcrumbs, preferably whole-wheat
- 1 small clove garlic, minced
- 8 tablespoons grated Parmesan cheese, divided
- 3 tablespoons finely chopped fresh parsley
- 3 large egg yolks
- 1 large egg
- ½ teaspoon ground pepper
- ¼ teaspoon salt
- 1 (9 ounce) package fresh tagliatelle or linguine
- 8 cups baby spinach
- 1 cup peas (fresh or frozen)

Directions

1. Put 10 cups of water in a large pot and bring to a boil over high heat.

2. Meanwhile, heat oil in a large skillet over medium-high heat. Add breadcrumbs and garlic; cook, stirring frequently, until toasted, about 2 minutes. Transfer to a small bowl and stir in 2 tablespoons Parmesan and parsley. Set aside.

3. Whisk the remaining 6 tablespoons Parmesan, egg yolks, egg, pepper and salt in a medium bowl.

4. Cook pasta in the boiling water, stirring occasionally, for 1 minute. Add spinach and peas and cook until the pasta is tender, about 1 minute more. Reserve 1/4 cup of the cooking water. Drain and place in a large bowl.

5. Slowly whisk the reserved cooking water into the egg mixture. Gradually add the mixture to

the pasta, tossing with tongs to combine. Serve topped with the reserved breadcrumb mixture.

Prep Time: 15 mins

Total Time: 40 mins

Servings: 6

Ingredients

- 2 tablespoons extra-virgin olive oil
- 3 cups fresh or frozen chopped onion, carrot and celery mix
- 4 cloves garlic, chopped
- 4 cups low-sodium vegetable or chicken broth
- 1 ½ cups green or brown lentils
- 1 (15-ounce) can unsalted diced tomatoes, undrained
- 2 teaspoons finely chopped fresh thyme
- ½ teaspoon salt
- ½ teaspoon ground pepper
- ½ teaspoon crushed red pepper
- ½ cup grated Parmesan cheese

- Parmesan rind (optional)
- 3 cups packed roughly chopped lacinato kale
- 1 ½ tablespoons red-wine vinegar
- Chopped fresh flat-leaf parsley for garnish

Directions

1. Heat oil in a Dutch oven or large pot over medium heat. Add onion, carrot and celery mix; cook, stirring occasionally, until softened, 6 to 10 minutes. Add garlic; cook, stirring often, until fragrant, about 30 seconds.

2. Stir in broth, lentils, tomatoes, thyme, salt, pepper, crushed red pepper and Parmesan rind, if using. Bring to a boil over medium-high heat. Reduce heat to medium-low; cover and cook, stirring occasionally, until the lentils are

almost tender, 15 to 25 minutes, adding water as needed to thin to desired consistency.

3. Stir in kale. Cook, covered, until the kale is tender, 5 to 10 minutes. Remove and discard the Parmesan rind, if using. Stir in vinegar. Divide the soup among 6 bowls; sprinkle with Parmesan. Garnish with parsley, if desired.

Prep Time: 15 mins

Total Time: 15 mins

Servings: 4

Ingredients

- ½ cup nonfat plain Greek yogurt

- ½ cup diced celery

- 2 tablespoons chopped fresh parsley

- 1 tablespoon lime juice

- 2 teaspoons mayonnaise

- 1 teaspoon Dijon mustard

- ⅛ teaspoon salt

- ⅛ teaspoon ground pepper

- 2 (5 ounce) cans salmon, drained, flaked, skin and bones removed

- 2 avocados

- Chopped chives for garnish

Directions

1. Combine yogurt, celery, parsley, lime juice, mayonnaise, mustard, salt, and pepper in a medium bowl; mix well. Add salmon and mix well.

2. Halve avocados lengthwise and remove pits. Scoop about 1 tablespoon flesh from each avocado half into a small bowl. Mash the scooped-out avocado flesh with a fork and stir into the salmon mixture.

3. Fill each avocado half with about 1/4 cup of the salmon mixture, mounding it on top of the avocado halves. Garnish with chives, if desired.

www.ingramcontent.com/pod-product-compliance
Lightning Source LLC
Chambersburg PA
CBHW061016260726
48661CB00005B/2211